I0096503

# TRAINING
## FOR A
# MAGICAL
# RACE

**This book belongs to:**

_____

ISBN: 979-8-9857816-0-1

# Table of Contents

# Race Details

## RACE

Race Name: _____

Distance(s): _____

Location: _____

Race Date(s): _____

Start Time: _____  Arrival Time: _____  Typical Race Size: _____

Course Description: _____

_____

_____

_____

_____

Average Temperature & Humidity: _____

Support (Before, During, & After): _____

_____

Charity/Team/Group: _____

Other Information: _____

_____

_____

## REGISTRATION

Date/Time/Method: _____

Cost: _____  Proof of Time: _____  Proof of Time Deadline: _____

Other Information: _____

_____

_____

## EXPO

Date(s) & Time(s): _____

Location: _____

Other Information: _____

_____

_____

# Training Goals & Plan

**Running Goals:**

☐ _____
☐ _____
☐ _____
☐ _____

**Strength Goals:**

☐ _____
☐ _____
☐ _____
☐ _____

**Nutrition Goals:**

☐ _____
☐ _____
☐ _____
☐ _____

**Other Goals:**

☐ _____
☐ _____
☐ _____
☐ _____

**How I Plan to Train:**_____

_____

_____

_____

_____

_____

_____

_____

_____

_____

# Training Weeks at a Glance

| Sun | Mon | Tue | Wed | Thu | Fri | Sat |
|-----|-----|-----|-----|-----|-----|-----|
|     |     |     |     |     |     |     |
|     |     |     |     |     |     |     |
|     |     |     |     |     |     |     |
|     |     |     |     |     |     |     |
|     |     |     |     |     |     |     |

Monthly Mileage: _____

| Sun | Mon | Tue | Wed | Thu | Fri | Sat |
|-----|-----|-----|-----|-----|-----|-----|
|     |     |     |     |     |     |     |
|     |     |     |     |     |     |     |
|     |     |     |     |     |     |     |
|     |     |     |     |     |     |     |
|     |     |     |     |     |     |     |
|     |     |     |     |     |     |     |

Monthly Mileage: _____

| Sun | Mon | Tue | Wed | Thu | Fri | Sat |
|-----|-----|-----|-----|-----|-----|-----|
|     |     |     |     |     |     |     |
|     |     |     |     |     |     |     |
|     |     |     |     |     |     |     |
|     |     |     |     |     |     |     |
|     |     |     |     |     |     |     |

Monthly Mileage: _____

| Sun | Mon | Tue | Wed | Thu | Fri | Sat |
|-----|-----|-----|-----|-----|-----|-----|
|     |     |     |     |     |     |     |
|     |     |     |     |     |     |     |
|     |     |     |     |     |     |     |
|     |     |     |     |     |     |     |
|     |     |     |     |     |     |     |
|     |     |     |     |     |     |     |

Monthly Mileage: _____

| Sun | Mon | Tue | Wed | Thu | Fri | Sat |
|-----|-----|-----|-----|-----|-----|-----|
|     |     |     |     |     |     |     |
|     |     |     |     |     |     |     |
|     |     |     |     |     |     |     |
|     |     |     |     |     |     |     |
|     |     |     |     |     |     |     |
|     |     |     |     |     |     |     |

Monthly Mileage: _____

| Sun | Mon | Tue | Wed | Thu | Fri | Sat |
|-----|-----|-----|-----|-----|-----|-----|
|     |     |     |     |     |     |     |
|     |     |     |     |     |     |     |
|     |     |     |     |     |     |     |
|     |     |     |     |     |     |     |
|     |     |     |     |     |     |     |
|     |     |     |     |     |     |     |

Monthly Mileage: _____

| Sun | Mon | Tue | Wed | Thu | Fri | Sat |
|-----|-----|-----|-----|-----|-----|-----|
|     |     |     |     |     |     |     |
|     |     |     |     |     |     |     |
|     |     |     |     |     |     |     |
|     |     |     |     |     |     |     |
|     |     |     |     |     |     |     |
|     |     |     |     |     |     |     |

Monthly Mileage: _____

| Sun | Mon | Tue | Wed | Thu | Fri | Sat |
|-----|-----|-----|-----|-----|-----|-----|
|     |     |     |     |     |     |     |
|     |     |     |     |     |     |     |
|     |     |     |     |     |     |     |
|     |     |     |     |     |     |     |
|     |     |     |     |     |     |     |
|     |     |     |     |     |     |     |

Monthly Mileage: _____

# Week #:

An amazing journey awaits!

Dates:

**How I'm Feeling:**

**Weekly Goals:**

| Date: | | Plan: | |
|---|---|---|---|
| **WORKOUT DESCRIPTION** | Run: | Cross-Train: | Strength: |
| | Time of Day: | Weather: | Cycle Day: |
| | Nutrition/Hydration: | | |
| | Notes: | | |

| Date: | | Plan: | |
|---|---|---|---|
| **WORKOUT DESCRIPTION** | Run: | Cross-Train: | Strength: |
| | Time of Day: | Weather: | Cycle Day: |
| | Nutrition/Hydration: | | |
| | Notes: | | |

| Date: | | Plan: | |
|---|---|---|---|
| **WORKOUT DESCRIPTION** | Run: | Cross-Train: | Strength: |
| | Time of Day: | Weather: | Cycle Day: |
| | Nutrition/Hydration: | | |
| | Notes: | | |

**Date:**          **Plan:**

**WORKOUT DESCRIPTION**

| Run: | Cross-Train: | Strength: |
|---|---|---|
| Time of Day: | Weather: | Cycle Day: |

Nutrition/Hydration:

Notes:

---

**Date:**          **Plan:**

**WORKOUT DESCRIPTION**

| Run: | Cross-Train: | Strength: |
|---|---|---|
| Time of Day: | Weather: | Cycle Day: |

Nutrition/Hydration:

Notes:

---

**Date:**          **Plan:**

**WORKOUT DESCRIPTION**

| Run: | Cross-Train: | Strength: |
|---|---|---|
| Time of Day: | Weather: | Cycle Day: |

Nutrition/Hydration:

Notes:

---

**Date:**          **Plan:**

**WORKOUT DESCRIPTION**

| Run: | Cross-Train: | Strength: |
|---|---|---|
| Time of Day: | Weather: | Cycle Day: |

Nutrition/Hydration:

Notes:          Weekly Mileage:

# Week #:　One week done! Way to go!　Dates:

**How I'm Feeling:**

**Weekly Goals:**

---

| WORKOUT DESCRIPTION | Date: | | Plan: | |
|---|---|---|---|---|
| | Run: | Cross-Train: | | Strength: |
| | Time of Day: | Weather: | | Cycle Day: |
| | Nutrition/Hydration: | | | |
| | Notes: | | | |

| WORKOUT DESCRIPTION | Date: | | Plan: | |
|---|---|---|---|---|
| | Run: | Cross-Train: | | Strength: |
| | Time of Day: | Weather: | | Cycle Day: |
| | Nutrition/Hydration: | | | |
| | Notes: | | | |

| WORKOUT DESCRIPTION | Date: | | Plan: | |
|---|---|---|---|---|
| | Run: | Cross-Train: | | Strength: |
| | Time of Day: | Weather: | | Cycle Day: |
| | Nutrition/Hydration: | | | |
| | Notes: | | | |

| WORKOUT DESCRIPTION | Date: | | Plan: | | |
|---|---|---|---|---|---|
| | Run: | | Cross-Train: | | Strength: |
| | Time of Day: | | Weather: | | Cycle Day: |
| | Nutrition/Hydration: | | | | |
| | Notes: | | | | |

| WORKOUT DESCRIPTION | Date: | | Plan: | | |
|---|---|---|---|---|---|
| | Run: | | Cross-Train: | | Strength: |
| | Time of Day: | | Weather: | | Cycle Day: |
| | Nutrition/Hydration: | | | | |
| | Notes: | | | | |

| WORKOUT DESCRIPTION | Date: | | Plan: | | |
|---|---|---|---|---|---|
| | Run: | | Cross-Train: | | Strength: |
| | Time of Day: | | Weather: | | Cycle Day: |
| | Nutrition/Hydration: | | | | |
| | Notes: | | | | |

| WORKOUT DESCRIPTION | Date: | | Plan: | | |
|---|---|---|---|---|---|
| | Run: | | Cross-Train: | | Strength: |
| | Time of Day: | | Weather: | | Cycle Day: |
| | Nutrition/Hydration: | | | | |
| | Notes: | | | | Weekly Mileage: |

# Week #:

Keep your easy days easy!

Dates:

**How I'm Feeling:**

**Weekly Goals:**

| Date: | | Plan: | |
|---|---|---|---|
| **WORKOUT DESCRIPTION** | Run: | Cross-Train: | Strength: |
| | Time of Day: | Weather: | Cycle Day: |
| | Nutrition/Hydration: | | |
| | Notes: | | |

| Date: | | Plan: | |
|---|---|---|---|
| **WORKOUT DESCRIPTION** | Run: | Cross-Train: | Strength: |
| | Time of Day: | Weather: | Cycle Day: |
| | Nutrition/Hydration: | | |
| | Notes: | | |

| Date: | | Plan: | |
|---|---|---|---|
| **WORKOUT DESCRIPTION** | Run: | Cross-Train: | Strength: |
| | Time of Day: | Weather: | Cycle Day: |
| | Nutrition/Hydration: | | |
| | Notes: | | |

**Date:**                **Plan:**

| WORKOUT DESCRIPTION | Run: | Cross-Train: | Strength: |
|---|---|---|---|
| | Time of Day: | Weather: | Cycle Day: |
| | Nutrition/Hydration: | | |
| | Notes: | | |

**Date:**                **Plan:**

| WORKOUT DESCRIPTION | Run: | Cross-Train: | Strength: |
|---|---|---|---|
| | Time of Day: | Weather: | Cycle Day: |
| | Nutrition/Hydration: | | |
| | Notes: | | |

**Date:**                **Plan:**

| WORKOUT DESCRIPTION | Run: | Cross-Train: | Strength: |
|---|---|---|---|
| | Time of Day: | Weather: | Cycle Day: |
| | Nutrition/Hydration: | | |
| | Notes: | | |

**Date:**                **Plan:**

| WORKOUT DESCRIPTION | Run: | Cross-Train: | Strength: |
|---|---|---|---|
| | Time of Day: | Weather: | Cycle Day: |
| | Nutrition/Hydration: | | |
| | Notes: | | Weekly Mileage: |

# Week #: Remember to warm up & cool down! | Dates:

**How I'm Feeling:**

**Weekly Goals:**

| WORKOUT DESCRIPTION | Date: | | Plan: | | |
|---|---|---|---|---|---|
| | Run: | | Cross-Train: | | Strength: |
| | Time of Day: | | Weather: | | Cycle Day: |
| | Nutrition/Hydration: | | | | |
| | Notes: | | | | |

| WORKOUT DESCRIPTION | Date: | | Plan: | | |
|---|---|---|---|---|---|
| | Run: | | Cross-Train: | | Strength: |
| | Time of Day: | | Weather: | | Cycle Day: |
| | Nutrition/Hydration: | | | | |
| | Notes: | | | | |

| WORKOUT DESCRIPTION | Date: | | Plan: | | |
|---|---|---|---|---|---|
| | Run: | | Cross-Train: | | Strength: |
| | Time of Day: | | Weather: | | Cycle Day: |
| | Nutrition/Hydration: | | | | |
| | Notes: | | | | |

| Date: | | Plan: | | |
|---|---|---|---|---|
| **WORKOUT DESCRIPTION** | Run: | Cross-Train: | | Strength: |
| | Time of Day: | Weather: | | Cycle Day: |
| | Nutrition/Hydration: | | | |
| | Notes: | | | |

| Date: | | Plan: | | |
|---|---|---|---|---|
| **WORKOUT DESCRIPTION** | Run: | Cross-Train: | | Strength: |
| | Time of Day: | Weather: | | Cycle Day: |
| | Nutrition/Hydration: | | | |
| | Notes: | | | |

| Date: | | Plan: | | |
|---|---|---|---|---|
| **WORKOUT DESCRIPTION** | Run: | Cross-Train: | | Strength: |
| | Time of Day: | Weather: | | Cycle Day: |
| | Nutrition/Hydration: | | | |
| | Notes: | | | |

| Date: | | Plan: | | |
|---|---|---|---|---|
| **WORKOUT DESCRIPTION** | Run: | Cross-Train: | | Strength: |
| | Time of Day: | Weather: | | Cycle Day: |
| | Nutrition/Hydration: | | | |
| | Notes: | | | Weekly Mileage: |

# Week #:

You're doing great! Keep it up!

Dates:

**How I'm Feeling:**

**Weekly Goals:**

---

**Date:** | **Plan:**

WORKOUT DESCRIPTION

| Run: | Cross-Train: | Strength: |
|------|--------------|-----------|
| Time of Day: | Weather: | Cycle Day: |

Nutrition/Hydration:

Notes:

---

**Date:** | **Plan:**

WORKOUT DESCRIPTION

| Run: | Cross-Train: | Strength: |
|------|--------------|-----------|
| Time of Day: | Weather: | Cycle Day: |

Nutrition/Hydration:

Notes:

---

**Date:** | **Plan:**

WORKOUT DESCRIPTION

| Run: | Cross-Train: | Strength: |
|------|--------------|-----------|
| Time of Day: | Weather: | Cycle Day: |

Nutrition/Hydration:

Notes:

| | | | |
|---|---|---|---|
| **Date:** | | **Plan:** | |

**WORKOUT DESCRIPTION**

| Run: | Cross-Train: | Strength: |
|---|---|---|
| Time of Day: | Weather: | Cycle Day: |

| Nutrition/Hydration: |
|---|

| Notes: |
|---|

---

| | | | |
|---|---|---|---|
| **Date:** | | **Plan:** | |

**WORKOUT DESCRIPTION**

| Run: | Cross-Train: | Strength: |
|---|---|---|
| Time of Day: | Weather: | Cycle Day: |

| Nutrition/Hydration: |
|---|

| Notes: |
|---|

---

| | | | |
|---|---|---|---|
| **Date:** | | **Plan:** | |

**WORKOUT DESCRIPTION**

| Run: | Cross-Train: | Strength: |
|---|---|---|
| Time of Day: | Weather: | Cycle Day: |

| Nutrition/Hydration: |
|---|

| Notes: |
|---|

---

| | | | |
|---|---|---|---|
| **Date:** | | **Plan:** | |

**WORKOUT DESCRIPTION**

| Run: | Cross-Train: | Strength: |
|---|---|---|
| Time of Day: | Weather: | Cycle Day: |

| Nutrition/Hydration: |
|---|

| Notes: | Weekly Mileage: |
|---|---|

# Week #:

Remember to fuel your runs!

Dates:

**How I'm Feeling:**

**Weekly Goals:**

| Date: | | Plan: | | | |
|---|---|---|---|---|---|
| **WORKOUT DESCRIPTION** | Run: | | Cross-Train: | | Strength: |
| | Time of Day: | | Weather: | | Cycle Day: |
| | Nutrition/Hydration: | | | | |
| | Notes: | | | | |

| Date: | | Plan: | | | |
|---|---|---|---|---|---|
| **WORKOUT DESCRIPTION** | Run: | | Cross-Train: | | Strength: |
| | Time of Day: | | Weather: | | Cycle Day: |
| | Nutrition/Hydration: | | | | |
| | Notes: | | | | |

| Date: | | Plan: | | | |
|---|---|---|---|---|---|
| **WORKOUT DESCRIPTION** | Run: | | Cross-Train: | | Strength: |
| | Time of Day: | | Weather: | | Cycle Day: |
| | Nutrition/Hydration: | | | | |
| | Notes: | | | | |

| Date: | | Plan: | | | |
|---|---|---|---|---|---|
| **WORKOUT DESCRIPTION** | Run: | | Cross-Train: | | Strength: |
| | Time of Day: | | Weather: | | Cycle Day: |
| | Nutrition/Hydration: | | | | |
| | Notes: | | | | |

| Date: | | Plan: | | | |
|---|---|---|---|---|---|
| **WORKOUT DESCRIPTION** | Run: | | Cross-Train: | | Strength: |
| | Time of Day: | | Weather: | | Cycle Day: |
| | Nutrition/Hydration: | | | | |
| | Notes: | | | | |

| Date: | | Plan: | | | |
|---|---|---|---|---|---|
| **WORKOUT DESCRIPTION** | Run: | | Cross-Train: | | Strength: |
| | Time of Day: | | Weather: | | Cycle Day: |
| | Nutrition/Hydration: | | | | |
| | Notes: | | | | |

| Date: | | Plan: | | | |
|---|---|---|---|---|---|
| **WORKOUT DESCRIPTION** | Run: | | Cross-Train: | | Strength: |
| | Time of Day: | | Weather: | | Cycle Day: |
| | Nutrition/Hydration: | | | | |
| | Notes: | | | | Weekly Mileage: |

# Week #:
Focus on one run at a time!

Dates:

**How I'm Feeling:**

**Weekly Goals:**

| Date: | | Plan: | |
|---|---|---|---|
| **WORKOUT DESCRIPTION** | Run: | Cross-Train: | Strength: |
| | Time of Day: | Weather: | Cycle Day: |
| | Nutrition/Hydration: | | |
| | Notes: | | |

| Date: | | Plan: | |
|---|---|---|---|
| **WORKOUT DESCRIPTION** | Run: | Cross-Train: | Strength: |
| | Time of Day: | Weather: | Cycle Day: |
| | Nutrition/Hydration: | | |
| | Notes: | | |

| Date: | | Plan: | |
|---|---|---|---|
| **WORKOUT DESCRIPTION** | Run: | Cross-Train: | Strength: |
| | Time of Day: | Weather: | Cycle Day: |
| | Nutrition/Hydration: | | |
| | Notes: | | |

| Date: | | Plan: | | |
|---|---|---|---|---|
| **WORKOUT DESCRIPTION** | Run: | Cross-Train: | | Strength: |
| | Time of Day: | Weather: | | Cycle Day: |
| | Nutrition/Hydration: | | | |
| | Notes: | | | |

| Date: | | Plan: | | |
|---|---|---|---|---|
| **WORKOUT DESCRIPTION** | Run: | Cross-Train: | | Strength: |
| | Time of Day: | Weather: | | Cycle Day: |
| | Nutrition/Hydration: | | | |
| | Notes: | | | |

| Date: | | Plan: | | |
|---|---|---|---|---|
| **WORKOUT DESCRIPTION** | Run: | Cross-Train: | | Strength: |
| | Time of Day: | Weather: | | Cycle Day: |
| | Nutrition/Hydration: | | | |
| | Notes: | | | |

| Date: | | Plan: | | |
|---|---|---|---|---|
| **WORKOUT DESCRIPTION** | Run: | Cross-Train: | | Strength: |
| | Time of Day: | Weather: | | Cycle Day: |
| | Nutrition/Hydration: | | | |
| | Notes: | | | Weekly Mileage: |

# Week #:

Remember to hydrate!

Dates:

**How I'm Feeling:**

**Weekly Goals:**

| Date: | | Plan: | |
|---|---|---|---|
| **WORKOUT DESCRIPTION** | Run: | Cross-Train: | Strength: |
| | Time of Day: | Weather: | Cycle Day: |
| | Nutrition/Hydration: | | |
| | Notes: | | |

| Date: | | Plan: | |
|---|---|---|---|
| **WORKOUT DESCRIPTION** | Run: | Cross-Train: | Strength: |
| | Time of Day: | Weather: | Cycle Day: |
| | Nutrition/Hydration: | | |
| | Notes: | | |

| Date: | | Plan: | |
|---|---|---|---|
| **WORKOUT DESCRIPTION** | Run: | Cross-Train: | Strength: |
| | Time of Day: | Weather: | Cycle Day: |
| | Nutrition/Hydration: | | |
| | Notes: | | |

**Date:** **Plan:**

| WORKOUT DESCRIPTION | Run: | Cross-Train: | Strength: |
|---|---|---|---|
| | Time of Day: | Weather: | Cycle Day: |
| | Nutrition/Hydration: | | |
| | Notes: | | |

**Date:** **Plan:**

| WORKOUT DESCRIPTION | Run: | Cross-Train: | Strength: |
|---|---|---|---|
| | Time of Day: | Weather: | Cycle Day: |
| | Nutrition/Hydration: | | |
| | Notes: | | |

**Date:** **Plan:**

| WORKOUT DESCRIPTION | Run: | Cross-Train: | Strength: |
|---|---|---|---|
| | Time of Day: | Weather: | Cycle Day: |
| | Nutrition/Hydration: | | |
| | Notes: | | |

**Date:** **Plan:**

| WORKOUT DESCRIPTION | Run: | Cross-Train: | Strength: |
|---|---|---|---|
| | Time of Day: | Weather: | Cycle Day: |
| | Nutrition/Hydration: | | |
| | Notes: | | Weekly Mileage: |

# Week #:

Recovery leads to growth!

Dates:

**How I'm Feeling:**

**Weekly Goals:**

---

Date: | Plan:

**WORKOUT DESCRIPTION**

| Run: | Cross-Train: | Strength: |
|---|---|---|
| Time of Day: | Weather: | Cycle Day: |
| Nutrition/Hydration: | | |
| Notes: | | |

---

Date: | Plan:

**WORKOUT DESCRIPTION**

| Run: | Cross-Train: | Strength: |
|---|---|---|
| Time of Day: | Weather: | Cycle Day: |
| Nutrition/Hydration: | | |
| Notes: | | |

---

Date: | Plan:

**WORKOUT DESCRIPTION**

| Run: | Cross-Train: | Strength: |
|---|---|---|
| Time of Day: | Weather: | Cycle Day: |
| Nutrition/Hydration: | | |
| Notes: | | |

**WORKOUT DESCRIPTION**

Date: | Plan:

| Run: | Cross-Train: | Strength: |
|------|--------------|-----------|
| Time of Day: | Weather: | Cycle Day: |

Nutrition/Hydration:

Notes:

---

**WORKOUT DESCRIPTION**

Date: | Plan:

| Run: | Cross-Train: | Strength: |
|------|--------------|-----------|
| Time of Day: | Weather: | Cycle Day: |

Nutrition/Hydration:

Notes:

---

**WORKOUT DESCRIPTION**

Date: | Plan:

| Run: | Cross-Train: | Strength: |
|------|--------------|-----------|
| Time of Day: | Weather: | Cycle Day: |

Nutrition/Hydration:

Notes:

---

**WORKOUT DESCRIPTION**

Date: | Plan:

| Run: | Cross-Train: | Strength: |
|------|--------------|-----------|
| Time of Day: | Weather: | Cycle Day: |

Nutrition/Hydration:

Notes: | Weekly Mileage:

# Week #:

You are strong!

Dates:

**How I'm Feeling:**

**Weekly Goals:**

| Date: | | Plan: | | |
|---|---|---|---|---|
| **WORKOUT DESCRIPTION** | Run: | Cross-Train: | | Strength: |
| | Time of Day: | Weather: | | Cycle Day: |
| | Nutrition/Hydration: | | | |
| | Notes: | | | |

| Date: | | Plan: | | |
|---|---|---|---|---|
| **WORKOUT DESCRIPTION** | Run: | Cross-Train: | | Strength: |
| | Time of Day: | Weather: | | Cycle Day: |
| | Nutrition/Hydration: | | | |
| | Notes: | | | |

| Date: | | Plan: | | |
|---|---|---|---|---|
| **WORKOUT DESCRIPTION** | Run: | Cross-Train: | | Strength: |
| | Time of Day: | Weather: | | Cycle Day: |
| | Nutrition/Hydration: | | | |
| | Notes: | | | |

**Date:**                  **Plan:**

| WORKOUT DESCRIPTION | Run: | Cross-Train: | Strength: |
|---|---|---|---|
| | Time of Day: | Weather: | Cycle Day: |
| | Nutrition/Hydration: | | |
| | Notes: | | |

**Date:**                  **Plan:**

| WORKOUT DESCRIPTION | Run: | Cross-Train: | Strength: |
|---|---|---|---|
| | Time of Day: | Weather: | Cycle Day: |
| | Nutrition/Hydration: | | |
| | Notes: | | |

**Date:**                  **Plan:**

| WORKOUT DESCRIPTION | Run: | Cross-Train: | Strength: |
|---|---|---|---|
| | Time of Day: | Weather: | Cycle Day: |
| | Nutrition/Hydration: | | |
| | Notes: | | |

**Date:**                  **Plan:**

| WORKOUT DESCRIPTION | Run: | Cross-Train: | Strength: |
|---|---|---|---|
| | Time of Day: | Weather: | Cycle Day: |
| | Nutrition/Hydration: | | |
| | Notes: | | Weekly Mileage: |

# Week #:

Activate those glutes!

Dates:

**How I'm Feeling:**

**Weekly Goals:**

---

Date: | Plan:

| WORKOUT DESCRIPTION | Run: | Cross-Train: | Strength: |
|---|---|---|---|
| | Time of Day: | Weather: | Cycle Day: |
| | Nutrition/Hydration: | | |
| | Notes: | | |

---

Date: | Plan:

| WORKOUT DESCRIPTION | Run: | Cross-Train: | Strength: |
|---|---|---|---|
| | Time of Day: | Weather: | Cycle Day: |
| | Nutrition/Hydration: | | |
| | Notes: | | |

---

Date: | Plan:

| WORKOUT DESCRIPTION | Run: | Cross-Train: | Strength: |
|---|---|---|---|
| | Time of Day: | Weather: | Cycle Day: |
| | Nutrition/Hydration: | | |
| | Notes: | | |

**WORKOUT DESCRIPTION**

| Date: | Plan: | |
|---|---|---|
| Run: | Cross-Train: | Strength: |
| Time of Day: | Weather: | Cycle Day: |
| Nutrition/Hydration: | | |
| Notes: | | |

**WORKOUT DESCRIPTION**

| Date: | Plan: | |
|---|---|---|
| Run: | Cross-Train: | Strength: |
| Time of Day: | Weather: | Cycle Day: |
| Nutrition/Hydration: | | |
| Notes: | | |

**WORKOUT DESCRIPTION**

| Date: | Plan: | |
|---|---|---|
| Run: | Cross-Train: | Strength: |
| Time of Day: | Weather: | Cycle Day: |
| Nutrition/Hydration: | | |
| Notes: | | |

**WORKOUT DESCRIPTION**

| Date: | Plan: | |
|---|---|---|
| Run: | Cross-Train: | Strength: |
| Time of Day: | Weather: | Cycle Day: |
| Nutrition/Hydration: | | |
| Notes: | | Weekly Mileage: |

# Week #:

Tough runs call for tunes!

Dates:

**How I'm Feeling:**

**Weekly Goals:**

| Date: | | Plan: | |
|---|---|---|---|
| **WORKOUT DESCRIPTION** | Run: | Cross-Train: | Strength: |
| | Time of Day: | Weather: | Cycle Day: |
| | Nutrition/Hydration: | | |
| | Notes: | | |

| Date: | | Plan: | |
|---|---|---|---|
| **WORKOUT DESCRIPTION** | Run: | Cross-Train: | Strength: |
| | Time of Day: | Weather: | Cycle Day: |
| | Nutrition/Hydration: | | |
| | Notes: | | |

| Date: | | Plan: | |
|---|---|---|---|
| **WORKOUT DESCRIPTION** | Run: | Cross-Train: | Strength: |
| | Time of Day: | Weather: | Cycle Day: |
| | Nutrition/Hydration: | | |
| | Notes: | | |

**Date:**                                   **Plan:**

WORKOUT DESCRIPTION

| Run: | Cross-Train: | Strength: |
|---|---|---|
| **Time of Day:** | **Weather:** | **Cycle Day:** |

**Nutrition/Hydration:**

**Notes:**

---

**Date:**                                   **Plan:**

WORKOUT DESCRIPTION

| Run: | Cross-Train: | Strength: |
|---|---|---|
| **Time of Day:** | **Weather:** | **Cycle Day:** |

**Nutrition/Hydration:**

**Notes:**

---

**Date:**                                   **Plan:**

WORKOUT DESCRIPTION

| Run: | Cross-Train: | Strength: |
|---|---|---|
| **Time of Day:** | **Weather:** | **Cycle Day:** |

**Nutrition/Hydration:**

**Notes:**

---

**Date:**                                   **Plan:**

WORKOUT DESCRIPTION

| Run: | Cross-Train: | Strength: |
|---|---|---|
| **Time of Day:** | **Weather:** | **Cycle Day:** |

**Nutrition/Hydration:**

**Notes:**                                                                      **Weekly Mileage:**

# Week #:

Test your fueling plan!

Dates:

**How I'm Feeling:**

**Weekly Goals:**

---

| Date: | | Plan: | | |
|---|---|---|---|---|
| **WORKOUT DESCRIPTION** | Run: | Cross-Train: | | Strength: |
| | Time of Day: | Weather: | | Cycle Day: |
| | Nutrition/Hydration: | | | |
| | Notes: | | | |

| Date: | | Plan: | | |
|---|---|---|---|---|
| **WORKOUT DESCRIPTION** | Run: | Cross-Train: | | Strength: |
| | Time of Day: | Weather: | | Cycle Day: |
| | Nutrition/Hydration: | | | |
| | Notes: | | | |

| Date: | | Plan: | | |
|---|---|---|---|---|
| **WORKOUT DESCRIPTION** | Run: | Cross-Train: | | Strength: |
| | Time of Day: | Weather: | | Cycle Day: |
| | Nutrition/Hydration: | | | |
| | Notes: | | | |

**WORKOUT DESCRIPTION**

| Date: | Plan: | |
|---|---|---|
| Run: | Cross-Train: | Strength: |
| Time of Day: | Weather: | Cycle Day: |
| Nutrition/Hydration: | | |
| Notes: | | |

| Date: | Plan: | |
|---|---|---|
| Run: | Cross-Train: | Strength: |
| Time of Day: | Weather: | Cycle Day: |
| Nutrition/Hydration: | | |
| Notes: | | |

| Date: | Plan: | |
|---|---|---|
| Run: | Cross-Train: | Strength: |
| Time of Day: | Weather: | Cycle Day: |
| Nutrition/Hydration: | | |
| Notes: | | |

| Date: | Plan: | |
|---|---|---|
| Run: | Cross-Train: | Strength: |
| Time of Day: | Weather: | Cycle Day: |
| Nutrition/Hydration: | | |
| Notes: | | Weekly Mileage: |

# Week #:

Test your race day outfit!

Dates:

**How I'm Feeling:**

**Weekly Goals:**

| Date: | | Plan: | |
|---|---|---|---|
| **WORKOUT DESCRIPTION** | Run: | Cross-Train: | Strength: |
| | Time of Day: | Weather: | Cycle Day: |
| | Nutrition/Hydration: | | |
| | Notes: | | |

| Date: | | Plan: | |
|---|---|---|---|
| **WORKOUT DESCRIPTION** | Run: | Cross-Train: | Strength: |
| | Time of Day: | Weather: | Cycle Day: |
| | Nutrition/Hydration: | | |
| | Notes: | | |

| Date: | | Plan: | |
|---|---|---|---|
| **WORKOUT DESCRIPTION** | Run: | Cross-Train: | Strength: |
| | Time of Day: | Weather: | Cycle Day: |
| | Nutrition/Hydration: | | |
| | Notes: | | |

**Date:**              **Plan:**

**WORKOUT DESCRIPTION**

| Run: | Cross-Train: | Strength: |
|---|---|---|
| Time of Day: | Weather: | Cycle Day: |

Nutrition/Hydration:

Notes:

---

**Date:**              **Plan:**

**WORKOUT DESCRIPTION**

| Run: | Cross-Train: | Strength: |
|---|---|---|
| Time of Day: | Weather: | Cycle Day: |

Nutrition/Hydration:

Notes:

---

**Date:**              **Plan:**

**WORKOUT DESCRIPTION**

| Run: | Cross-Train: | Strength: |
|---|---|---|
| Time of Day: | Weather: | Cycle Day: |

Nutrition/Hydration:

Notes:

---

**Date:**              **Plan:**

**WORKOUT DESCRIPTION**

| Run: | Cross-Train: | Strength: |
|---|---|---|
| Time of Day: | Weather: | Cycle Day: |

Nutrition/Hydration:

Notes:                          **Weekly Mileage:**

# Week #:

You're getting it done!

Dates:

**How I'm Feeling:**

**Weekly Goals:**

---

Date: | Plan:

WORKOUT DESCRIPTION

| Run: | Cross-Train: | Strength: |
|---|---|---|
| Time of Day: | Weather: | Cycle Day: |

Nutrition/Hydration:

Notes:

---

Date: | Plan:

| Run: | Cross-Train: | Strength: |
|---|---|---|
| Time of Day: | Weather: | Cycle Day: |

Nutrition/Hydration:

Notes:

---

Date: | Plan:

| Run: | Cross-Train: | Strength: |
|---|---|---|
| Time of Day: | Weather: | Cycle Day: |

Nutrition/Hydration:

Notes:

| Date: | | Plan: | | |
|---|---|---|---|---|
| **WORKOUT DESCRIPTION** | Run: | Cross-Train: | | Strength: |
| | Time of Day: | Weather: | | Cycle Day: |
| | Nutrition/Hydration: | | | |
| | Notes: | | | |

| Date: | | Plan: | | |
|---|---|---|---|---|
| **WORKOUT DESCRIPTION** | Run: | Cross-Train: | | Strength: |
| | Time of Day: | Weather: | | Cycle Day: |
| | Nutrition/Hydration: | | | |
| | Notes: | | | |

| Date: | | Plan: | | |
|---|---|---|---|---|
| **WORKOUT DESCRIPTION** | Run: | Cross-Train: | | Strength: |
| | Time of Day: | Weather: | | Cycle Day: |
| | Nutrition/Hydration: | | | |
| | Notes: | | | |

| Date: | | Plan: | | |
|---|---|---|---|---|
| **WORKOUT DESCRIPTION** | Run: | Cross-Train: | | Strength: |
| | Time of Day: | Weather: | | Cycle Day: |
| | Nutrition/Hydration: | | | |
| | Notes: | | | Weekly Mileage: |

# Week #:  Sleep is important! Get enough!  Dates:

**How I'm Feeling:**

**Weekly Goals:**

| Date: | | Plan: | | |
|---|---|---|---|---|
| **WORKOUT DESCRIPTION** | Run: | Cross-Train: | | Strength: |
| | Time of Day: | Weather: | | Cycle Day: |
| | Nutrition/Hydration: | | | |
| | Notes: | | | |

| Date: | | Plan: | | |
|---|---|---|---|---|
| **WORKOUT DESCRIPTION** | Run: | Cross-Train: | | Strength: |
| | Time of Day: | Weather: | | Cycle Day: |
| | Nutrition/Hydration: | | | |
| | Notes: | | | |

| Date: | | Plan: | | |
|---|---|---|---|---|
| **WORKOUT DESCRIPTION** | Run: | Cross-Train: | | Strength: |
| | Time of Day: | Weather: | | Cycle Day: |
| | Nutrition/Hydration: | | | |
| | Notes: | | | |

**WORKOUT DESCRIPTION**

Date: | Plan:

| Run: | Cross-Train: | Strength: |
| Time of Day: | Weather: | Cycle Day: |

Nutrition/Hydration:

Notes:

---

**WORKOUT DESCRIPTION**

Date: | Plan:

| Run: | Cross-Train: | Strength: |
| Time of Day: | Weather: | Cycle Day: |

Nutrition/Hydration:

Notes:

---

**WORKOUT DESCRIPTION**

Date: | Plan:

| Run: | Cross-Train: | Strength: |
| Time of Day: | Weather: | Cycle Day: |

Nutrition/Hydration:

Notes:

---

**WORKOUT DESCRIPTION**

Date: | Plan:

| Run: | Cross-Train: | Strength: |
| Time of Day: | Weather: | Cycle Day: |

Nutrition/Hydration:

Notes: | Weekly Mileage:

| Week #: | Refuel after your run! | Dates: |
|---|---|---|

**How I'm Feeling:**

**Weekly Goals:**

---

| Date: | | Plan: | |
|---|---|---|---|

<table>
<tr><td rowspan="5" style="writing-mode:vertical">WORKOUT DESCRIPTION</td><td>Run:</td><td>Cross-Train:</td><td>Strength:</td></tr>
<tr><td>Time of Day:</td><td>Weather:</td><td>Cycle Day:</td></tr>
<tr><td colspan="3">Nutrition/Hydration:</td></tr>
<tr><td colspan="3">Notes:</td></tr>
</table>

---

| Date: | | Plan: | |
|---|---|---|---|

<table>
<tr><td rowspan="5" style="writing-mode:vertical">WORKOUT DESCRIPTION</td><td>Run:</td><td>Cross-Train:</td><td>Strength:</td></tr>
<tr><td>Time of Day:</td><td>Weather:</td><td>Cycle Day:</td></tr>
<tr><td colspan="3">Nutrition/Hydration:</td></tr>
<tr><td colspan="3">Notes:</td></tr>
</table>

---

| Date: | | Plan: | |
|---|---|---|---|

<table>
<tr><td rowspan="5" style="writing-mode:vertical">WORKOUT DESCRIPTION</td><td>Run:</td><td>Cross-Train:</td><td>Strength:</td></tr>
<tr><td>Time of Day:</td><td>Weather:</td><td>Cycle Day:</td></tr>
<tr><td colspan="3">Nutrition/Hydration:</td></tr>
<tr><td colspan="3">Notes:</td></tr>
</table>

**Date:** | **Plan:**

| WORKOUT DESCRIPTION | Run: | Cross-Train: | Strength: |
|---|---|---|---|
| | Time of Day: | Weather: | Cycle Day: |
| | Nutrition/Hydration: | | |
| | Notes: | | |

**Date:** | **Plan:**

| WORKOUT DESCRIPTION | Run: | Cross-Train: | Strength: |
|---|---|---|---|
| | Time of Day: | Weather: | Cycle Day: |
| | Nutrition/Hydration: | | |
| | Notes: | | |

**Date:** | **Plan:**

| WORKOUT DESCRIPTION | Run: | Cross-Train: | Strength: |
|---|---|---|---|
| | Time of Day: | Weather: | Cycle Day: |
| | Nutrition/Hydration: | | |
| | Notes: | | |

**Date:** | **Plan:**

| WORKOUT DESCRIPTION | Run: | Cross-Train: | Strength: |
|---|---|---|---|
| | Time of Day: | Weather: | Cycle Day: |
| | Nutrition/Hydration: | | |
| | Notes: | | Weekly Mileage: |

# Week #:

You've got this!

Dates:

**How I'm Feeling:**

**Weekly Goals:**

---

Date: | Plan:

| WORKOUT DESCRIPTION | Run: | Cross-Train: | Strength: |
|---|---|---|---|
| | Time of Day: | Weather: | Cycle Day: |
| | Nutrition/Hydration: | | |
| | Notes: | | |

---

Date: | Plan:

| WORKOUT DESCRIPTION | Run: | Cross-Train: | Strength: |
|---|---|---|---|
| | Time of Day: | Weather: | Cycle Day: |
| | Nutrition/Hydration: | | |
| | Notes: | | |

---

Date: | Plan:

| WORKOUT DESCRIPTION | Run: | Cross-Train: | Strength: |
|---|---|---|---|
| | Time of Day: | Weather: | Cycle Day: |
| | Nutrition/Hydration: | | |
| | Notes: | | |

| | | Plan: | | |
|---|---|---|---|---|
| Date: | | Plan: | | |

**WORKOUT DESCRIPTION**

| Run: | Cross-Train: | Strength: |
|---|---|---|
| Time of Day: | Weather: | Cycle Day: |
| Nutrition/Hydration: | | |
| Notes: | | |

---

| Date: | | Plan: | | |
|---|---|---|---|---|

**WORKOUT DESCRIPTION**

| Run: | Cross-Train: | Strength: |
|---|---|---|
| Time of Day: | Weather: | Cycle Day: |
| Nutrition/Hydration: | | |
| Notes: | | |

---

| Date: | | Plan: | | |
|---|---|---|---|---|

**WORKOUT DESCRIPTION**

| Run: | Cross-Train: | Strength: |
|---|---|---|
| Time of Day: | Weather: | Cycle Day: |
| Nutrition/Hydration: | | |
| Notes: | | |

---

| Date: | | Plan: | | |
|---|---|---|---|---|

**WORKOUT DESCRIPTION**

| Run: | Cross-Train: | Strength: |
|---|---|---|
| Time of Day: | Weather: | Cycle Day: |
| Nutrition/Hydration: | | |
| Notes: | | Weekly Mileage: |

# Week #:

Remember to smile!

Dates:

**How I'm Feeling:**

**Weekly Goals:**

---

Date: | | Plan:
---|---|---

| | Run: | Cross-Train: | Strength: |
|---|---|---|---|
| **WORKOUT DESCRIPTION** | Time of Day: | Weather: | Cycle Day: |
| | Nutrition/Hydration: | | |
| | Notes: | | |

---

Date: | | Plan:
---|---|---

| | Run: | Cross-Train: | Strength: |
|---|---|---|---|
| **WORKOUT DESCRIPTION** | Time of Day: | Weather: | Cycle Day: |
| | Nutrition/Hydration: | | |
| | Notes: | | |

---

Date: | | Plan:
---|---|---

| | Run: | Cross-Train: | Strength: |
|---|---|---|---|
| **WORKOUT DESCRIPTION** | Time of Day: | Weather: | Cycle Day: |
| | Nutrition/Hydration: | | |
| | Notes: | | |

| | Date: | | Plan: | | |
|---|---|---|---|---|---|
| **WORKOUT DESCRIPTION** | Run: | | Cross-Train: | | Strength: |
| | Time of Day: | | Weather: | | Cycle Day: |
| | Nutrition/Hydration: | | | | |
| | Notes: | | | | |

| | Date: | | Plan: | | |
|---|---|---|---|---|---|
| **WORKOUT DESCRIPTION** | Run: | | Cross-Train: | | Strength: |
| | Time of Day: | | Weather: | | Cycle Day: |
| | Nutrition/Hydration: | | | | |
| | Notes: | | | | |

| | Date: | | Plan: | | |
|---|---|---|---|---|---|
| **WORKOUT DESCRIPTION** | Run: | | Cross-Train: | | Strength: |
| | Time of Day: | | Weather: | | Cycle Day: |
| | Nutrition/Hydration: | | | | |
| | Notes: | | | | |

| | Date: | | Plan: | | |
|---|---|---|---|---|---|
| **WORKOUT DESCRIPTION** | Run: | | Cross-Train: | | Strength: |
| | Time of Day: | | Weather: | | Cycle Day: |
| | Nutrition/Hydration: | | | | |
| | Notes: | | | | Weekly Mileage: |

# Week #:

You've come so far!

Dates:

**How I'm Feeling:**

**Weekly Goals:**

---

**Date:** | **Plan:**

| WORKOUT DESCRIPTION | Run: | Cross-Train: | Strength: |
|---|---|---|---|
| | Time of Day: | Weather: | Cycle Day: |
| | Nutrition/Hydration: | | |
| | Notes: | | |

---

**Date:** | **Plan:**

| WORKOUT DESCRIPTION | Run: | Cross-Train: | Strength: |
|---|---|---|---|
| | Time of Day: | Weather: | Cycle Day: |
| | Nutrition/Hydration: | | |
| | Notes: | | |

---

**Date:** | **Plan:**

| WORKOUT DESCRIPTION | Run: | Cross-Train: | Strength: |
|---|---|---|---|
| | Time of Day: | Weather: | Cycle Day: |
| | Nutrition/Hydration: | | |
| | Notes: | | |

| Date: | Plan: | |
|---|---|---|
| **WORKOUT DESCRIPTION** Run: | Cross-Train: | Strength: |
| Time of Day: | Weather: | Cycle Day: |
| Nutrition/Hydration: | | |
| Notes: | | |

| Date: | Plan: | |
|---|---|---|
| **WORKOUT DESCRIPTION** Run: | Cross-Train: | Strength: |
| Time of Day: | Weather: | Cycle Day: |
| Nutrition/Hydration: | | |
| Notes: | | |

| Date: | Plan: | |
|---|---|---|
| **WORKOUT DESCRIPTION** Run: | Cross-Train: | Strength: |
| Time of Day: | Weather: | Cycle Day: |
| Nutrition/Hydration: | | |
| Notes: | | |

| Date: | Plan: | |
|---|---|---|
| **WORKOUT DESCRIPTION** Run: | Cross-Train: | Strength: |
| Time of Day: | Weather: | Cycle Day: |
| Nutrition/Hydration: | | |
| Notes: | | Weekly Mileage: |

# Week #:

Keep stepping forward!

Dates:

**How I'm Feeling:**

**Weekly Goals:**

---

Date: | Plan:

<table>
<tr><td rowspan="5" style="writing-mode: vertical-rl;">WORKOUT DESCRIPTION</td><td>Run:</td><td>Cross-Train:</td><td>Strength:</td></tr>
<tr><td>Time of Day:</td><td>Weather:</td><td>Cycle Day:</td></tr>
<tr><td colspan="3">Nutrition/Hydration:</td></tr>
<tr><td colspan="3">Notes:</td></tr>
</table>

---

Date: | Plan:

<table>
<tr><td rowspan="5" style="writing-mode: vertical-rl;">WORKOUT DESCRIPTION</td><td>Run:</td><td>Cross-Train:</td><td>Strength:</td></tr>
<tr><td>Time of Day:</td><td>Weather:</td><td>Cycle Day:</td></tr>
<tr><td colspan="3">Nutrition/Hydration:</td></tr>
<tr><td colspan="3">Notes:</td></tr>
</table>

---

Date: | Plan:

<table>
<tr><td rowspan="5" style="writing-mode: vertical-rl;">WORKOUT DESCRIPTION</td><td>Run:</td><td>Cross-Train:</td><td>Strength:</td></tr>
<tr><td>Time of Day:</td><td>Weather:</td><td>Cycle Day:</td></tr>
<tr><td colspan="3">Nutrition/Hydration:</td></tr>
<tr><td colspan="3">Notes:</td></tr>
</table>

| | Date: | | Plan: | | |
|---|---|---|---|---|---|
| **WORKOUT DESCRIPTION** | Run: | | Cross-Train: | | Strength: |
| | Time of Day: | | Weather: | | Cycle Day: |
| | Nutrition/Hydration: | | | | |
| | Notes: | | | | |

| | Date: | | Plan: | | |
|---|---|---|---|---|---|
| **WORKOUT DESCRIPTION** | Run: | | Cross-Train: | | Strength: |
| | Time of Day: | | Weather: | | Cycle Day: |
| | Nutrition/Hydration: | | | | |
| | Notes: | | | | |

| | Date: | | Plan: | | |
|---|---|---|---|---|---|
| **WORKOUT DESCRIPTION** | Run: | | Cross-Train: | | Strength: |
| | Time of Day: | | Weather: | | Cycle Day: |
| | Nutrition/Hydration: | | | | |
| | Notes: | | | | |

| | Date: | | Plan: | | |
|---|---|---|---|---|---|
| **WORKOUT DESCRIPTION** | Run: | | Cross-Train: | | Strength: |
| | Time of Day: | | Weather: | | Cycle Day: |
| | Nutrition/Hydration: | | | | |
| | Notes: | | | | Weekly Mileage: |

# Week #:

You can do hard things!

**Dates:**

**How I'm Feeling:**

**Weekly Goals:**

| Date: | | Plan: | |
|---|---|---|---|
| **WORKOUT DESCRIPTION** | Run: | Cross-Train: | Strength: |
| | Time of Day: | Weather: | Cycle Day: |
| | Nutrition/Hydration: | | |
| | Notes: | | |

| Date: | | Plan: | |
|---|---|---|---|
| **WORKOUT DESCRIPTION** | Run: | Cross-Train: | Strength: |
| | Time of Day: | Weather: | Cycle Day: |
| | Nutrition/Hydration: | | |
| | Notes: | | |

| Date: | | Plan: | |
|---|---|---|---|
| **WORKOUT DESCRIPTION** | Run: | Cross-Train: | Strength: |
| | Time of Day: | Weather: | Cycle Day: |
| | Nutrition/Hydration: | | |
| | Notes: | | |

**Date:** | **Plan:**

**WORKOUT DESCRIPTION**

| Run: | Cross-Train: | Strength: |
|---|---|---|
| Time of Day: | Weather: | Cycle Day: |

Nutrition/Hydration:

Notes:

---

**Date:** | **Plan:**

**WORKOUT DESCRIPTION**

| Run: | Cross-Train: | Strength: |
|---|---|---|
| Time of Day: | Weather: | Cycle Day: |

Nutrition/Hydration:

Notes:

---

**Date:** | **Plan:**

**WORKOUT DESCRIPTION**

| Run: | Cross-Train: | Strength: |
|---|---|---|
| Time of Day: | Weather: | Cycle Day: |

Nutrition/Hydration:

Notes:

---

**Date:** | **Plan:**

**WORKOUT DESCRIPTION**

| Run: | Cross-Train: | Strength: |
|---|---|---|
| Time of Day: | Weather: | Cycle Day: |

Nutrition/Hydration:

Notes: | | Weekly Mileage:

# Week #:                 Some runs are tough!                 Dates:

**How I'm Feeling:**

**Weekly Goals:**

| Date: | | Plan: | | |
|---|---|---|---|---|
| **WORKOUT DESCRIPTION** | Run: | Cross-Train: | | Strength: |
| | Time of Day: | Weather: | | Cycle Day: |
| | Nutrition/Hydration: | | | |
| | Notes: | | | |

| Date: | | Plan: | | |
|---|---|---|---|---|
| **WORKOUT DESCRIPTION** | Run: | Cross-Train: | | Strength: |
| | Time of Day: | Weather: | | Cycle Day: |
| | Nutrition/Hydration: | | | |
| | Notes: | | | |

| Date: | | Plan: | | |
|---|---|---|---|---|
| **WORKOUT DESCRIPTION** | Run: | Cross-Train: | | Strength: |
| | Time of Day: | Weather: | | Cycle Day: |
| | Nutrition/Hydration: | | | |
| | Notes: | | | |

| | Date: | | Plan: | | |
|---|---|---|---|---|---|
| **WORKOUT DESCRIPTION** | Run: | | Cross-Train: | | Strength: |
| | Time of Day: | | Weather: | | Cycle Day: |
| | Nutrition/Hydration: | | | | |
| | Notes: | | | | |

| | Date: | | Plan: | | |
|---|---|---|---|---|---|
| **WORKOUT DESCRIPTION** | Run: | | Cross-Train: | | Strength: |
| | Time of Day: | | Weather: | | Cycle Day: |
| | Nutrition/Hydration: | | | | |
| | Notes: | | | | |

| | Date: | | Plan: | | |
|---|---|---|---|---|---|
| **WORKOUT DESCRIPTION** | Run: | | Cross-Train: | | Strength: |
| | Time of Day: | | Weather: | | Cycle Day: |
| | Nutrition/Hydration: | | | | |
| | Notes: | | | | |

| | Date: | | Plan: | | |
|---|---|---|---|---|---|
| **WORKOUT DESCRIPTION** | Run: | | Cross-Train: | | Strength: |
| | Time of Day: | | Weather: | | Cycle Day: |
| | Nutrition/Hydration: | | | | |
| | Notes: | | | | Weekly Mileage: |

# Week #:

Some runs are just for fun!

Dates:

**How I'm Feeling:**

**Weekly Goals:**

| Date: | | Plan: | | |
|---|---|---|---|---|
| **WORKOUT DESCRIPTION** | Run: | Cross-Train: | | Strength: |
| | Time of Day: | Weather: | | Cycle Day: |
| | Nutrition/Hydration: | | | |
| | Notes: | | | |

| Date: | | Plan: | | |
|---|---|---|---|---|
| **WORKOUT DESCRIPTION** | Run: | Cross-Train: | | Strength: |
| | Time of Day: | Weather: | | Cycle Day: |
| | Nutrition/Hydration: | | | |
| | Notes: | | | |

| Date: | | Plan: | | |
|---|---|---|---|---|
| **WORKOUT DESCRIPTION** | Run: | Cross-Train: | | Strength: |
| | Time of Day: | Weather: | | Cycle Day: |
| | Nutrition/Hydration: | | | |
| | Notes: | | | |

| WORKOUT DESCRIPTION | Date: | | Plan: | | |
|---|---|---|---|---|---|
| | Run: | | Cross-Train: | | Strength: |
| | Time of Day: | | Weather: | | Cycle Day: |
| | Nutrition/Hydration: | | | | |
| | Notes: | | | | |

| WORKOUT DESCRIPTION | Date: | | Plan: | | |
|---|---|---|---|---|---|
| | Run: | | Cross-Train: | | Strength: |
| | Time of Day: | | Weather: | | Cycle Day: |
| | Nutrition/Hydration: | | | | |
| | Notes: | | | | |

| WORKOUT DESCRIPTION | Date: | | Plan: | | |
|---|---|---|---|---|---|
| | Run: | | Cross-Train: | | Strength: |
| | Time of Day: | | Weather: | | Cycle Day: |
| | Nutrition/Hydration: | | | | |
| | Notes: | | | | |

| WORKOUT DESCRIPTION | Date: | | Plan: | | |
|---|---|---|---|---|---|
| | Run: | | Cross-Train: | | Strength: |
| | Time of Day: | | Weather: | | Cycle Day: |
| | Nutrition/Hydration: | | | | |
| | Notes: | | | | Weekly Mileage: |

# Week #:

Keep going! You can do it!

**Dates:**

**How I'm Feeling:**

**Weekly Goals:**

| Date: | | Plan: | | |
|---|---|---|---|---|
| **WORKOUT DESCRIPTION** | Run: | Cross-Train: | | Strength: |
| | Time of Day: | Weather: | | Cycle Day: |
| | Nutrition/Hydration: | | | |
| | Notes: | | | |

| Date: | | Plan: | | |
|---|---|---|---|---|
| **WORKOUT DESCRIPTION** | Run: | Cross-Train: | | Strength: |
| | Time of Day: | Weather: | | Cycle Day: |
| | Nutrition/Hydration: | | | |
| | Notes: | | | |

| Date: | | Plan: | | |
|---|---|---|---|---|
| **WORKOUT DESCRIPTION** | Run: | Cross-Train: | | Strength: |
| | Time of Day: | Weather: | | Cycle Day: |
| | Nutrition/Hydration: | | | |
| | Notes: | | | |

| Date: | | Plan: | | |
|---|---|---|---|---|
| **WORKOUT DESCRIPTION** | Run: | Cross-Train: | | Strength: |
| | Time of Day: | Weather: | | Cycle Day: |
| | Nutrition/Hydration: | | | |
| | Notes: | | | |

| Date: | | Plan: | | |
|---|---|---|---|---|
| **WORKOUT DESCRIPTION** | Run: | Cross-Train: | | Strength: |
| | Time of Day: | Weather: | | Cycle Day: |
| | Nutrition/Hydration: | | | |
| | Notes: | | | |

| Date: | | Plan: | | |
|---|---|---|---|---|
| **WORKOUT DESCRIPTION** | Run: | Cross-Train: | | Strength: |
| | Time of Day: | Weather: | | Cycle Day: |
| | Nutrition/Hydration: | | | |
| | Notes: | | | |

| Date: | | Plan: | | |
|---|---|---|---|---|
| **WORKOUT DESCRIPTION** | Run: | Cross-Train: | | Strength: |
| | Time of Day: | Weather: | | Cycle Day: |
| | Nutrition/Hydration: | | | |
| | Notes: | | | Weekly Mileage: |

# Week #:

You are brave!

Dates:

**How I'm Feeling:**

**Weekly Goals:**

---

**Date:** | **Plan:**

WORKOUT DESCRIPTION

| Run: | Cross-Train: | Strength: |
|---|---|---|
| Time of Day: | Weather: | Cycle Day: |
| Nutrition/Hydration: | | |
| Notes: | | |

---

**Date:** | **Plan:**

WORKOUT DESCRIPTION

| Run: | Cross-Train: | Strength: |
|---|---|---|
| Time of Day: | Weather: | Cycle Day: |
| Nutrition/Hydration: | | |
| Notes: | | |

---

**Date:** | **Plan:**

WORKOUT DESCRIPTION

| Run: | Cross-Train: | Strength: |
|---|---|---|
| Time of Day: | Weather: | Cycle Day: |
| Nutrition/Hydration: | | |
| Notes: | | |

**Date:**        **Plan:**

| WORKOUT DESCRIPTION | Run: | Cross-Train: | Strength: |
|---|---|---|---|
| | Time of Day: | Weather: | Cycle Day: |
| | Nutrition/Hydration: | | |
| | Notes: | | |

**Date:**        **Plan:**

| WORKOUT DESCRIPTION | Run: | Cross-Train: | Strength: |
|---|---|---|---|
| | Time of Day: | Weather: | Cycle Day: |
| | Nutrition/Hydration: | | |
| | Notes: | | |

**Date:**        **Plan:**

| WORKOUT DESCRIPTION | Run: | Cross-Train: | Strength: |
|---|---|---|---|
| | Time of Day: | Weather: | Cycle Day: |
| | Nutrition/Hydration: | | |
| | Notes: | | |

**Date:**        **Plan:**

| WORKOUT DESCRIPTION | Run: | Cross-Train: | Strength: |
|---|---|---|---|
| | Time of Day: | Weather: | Cycle Day: |
| | Nutrition/Hydration: | | |
| | Notes: | | Weekly Mileage: |

# Week #:                    Let go of fear!                    Dates:

**How I'm Feeling:**

**Weekly Goals:**

| Date: | | Plan: | |
|---|---|---|---|
| **WORKOUT DESCRIPTION** | Run: | Cross-Train: | Strength: |
| | Time of Day: | Weather: | Cycle Day: |
| | Nutrition/Hydration: | | |
| | Notes: | | |

| Date: | | Plan: | |
|---|---|---|---|
| **WORKOUT DESCRIPTION** | Run: | Cross-Train: | Strength: |
| | Time of Day: | Weather: | Cycle Day: |
| | Nutrition/Hydration: | | |
| | Notes: | | |

| Date: | | Plan: | |
|---|---|---|---|
| **WORKOUT DESCRIPTION** | Run: | Cross-Train: | Strength: |
| | Time of Day: | Weather: | Cycle Day: |
| | Nutrition/Hydration: | | |
| | Notes: | | |

**WORKOUT DESCRIPTION**

| Date: | | Plan: | | |
|---|---|---|---|---|
| Run: | | Cross-Train: | | Strength: |
| Time of Day: | | Weather: | | Cycle Day: |
| Nutrition/Hydration: | | | | |
| Notes: | | | | |

**WORKOUT DESCRIPTION**

| Date: | | Plan: | | |
|---|---|---|---|---|
| Run: | | Cross-Train: | | Strength: |
| Time of Day: | | Weather: | | Cycle Day: |
| Nutrition/Hydration: | | | | |
| Notes: | | | | |

**WORKOUT DESCRIPTION**

| Date: | | Plan: | | |
|---|---|---|---|---|
| Run: | | Cross-Train: | | Strength: |
| Time of Day: | | Weather: | | Cycle Day: |
| Nutrition/Hydration: | | | | |
| Notes: | | | | |

**WORKOUT DESCRIPTION**

| Date: | | Plan: | | |
|---|---|---|---|---|
| Run: | | Cross-Train: | | Strength: |
| Time of Day: | | Weather: | | Cycle Day: |
| Nutrition/Hydration: | | | | |
| Notes: | | | | Weekly Mileage: |

# Week #:                    Stay focused!                    Dates:

**How I'm Feeling:**

**Weekly Goals:**

| Date: | Plan: | |
|---|---|---|
| **Run:** | **Cross-Train:** | **Strength:** |
| **Time of Day:** | **Weather:** | **Cycle Day:** |
| **Nutrition/Hydration:** | | |
| **Notes:** | | |

*WORKOUT DESCRIPTION*

| Date: | Plan: | |
|---|---|---|
| **Run:** | **Cross-Train:** | **Strength:** |
| **Time of Day:** | **Weather:** | **Cycle Day:** |
| **Nutrition/Hydration:** | | |
| **Notes:** | | |

*WORKOUT DESCRIPTION*

| Date: | Plan: | |
|---|---|---|
| **Run:** | **Cross-Train:** | **Strength:** |
| **Time of Day:** | **Weather:** | **Cycle Day:** |
| **Nutrition/Hydration:** | | |
| **Notes:** | | |

*WORKOUT DESCRIPTION*

| Date: | | Plan: | | | |
|---|---|---|---|---|---|
| **WORKOUT DESCRIPTION** | Run: | | Cross-Train: | | Strength: |
| | Time of Day: | | Weather: | | Cycle Day: |
| | Nutrition/Hydration: | | | | |
| | Notes: | | | | |

| Date: | | Plan: | | | |
|---|---|---|---|---|---|
| **WORKOUT DESCRIPTION** | Run: | | Cross-Train: | | Strength: |
| | Time of Day: | | Weather: | | Cycle Day: |
| | Nutrition/Hydration: | | | | |
| | Notes: | | | | |

| Date: | | Plan: | | | |
|---|---|---|---|---|---|
| **WORKOUT DESCRIPTION** | Run: | | Cross-Train: | | Strength: |
| | Time of Day: | | Weather: | | Cycle Day: |
| | Nutrition/Hydration: | | | | |
| | Notes: | | | | |

| Date: | | Plan: | | | |
|---|---|---|---|---|---|
| **WORKOUT DESCRIPTION** | Run: | | Cross-Train: | | Strength: |
| | Time of Day: | | Weather: | | Cycle Day: |
| | Nutrition/Hydration: | | | | |
| | Notes: | | | Weekly Mileage: | | |

# Week #:    Each day is a new beginning!    Dates:

**How I'm Feeling:**

**Weekly Goals:**

| Date: | | Plan: | |
|---|---|---|---|
| **WORKOUT DESCRIPTION** | Run: | Cross-Train: | Strength: |
| | Time of Day: | Weather: | Cycle Day: |
| | Nutrition/Hydration: | | |
| | Notes: | | |

| Date: | | Plan: | |
|---|---|---|---|
| **WORKOUT DESCRIPTION** | Run: | Cross-Train: | Strength: |
| | Time of Day: | Weather: | Cycle Day: |
| | Nutrition/Hydration: | | |
| | Notes: | | |

| Date: | | Plan: | |
|---|---|---|---|
| **WORKOUT DESCRIPTION** | Run: | Cross-Train: | Strength: |
| | Time of Day: | Weather: | Cycle Day: |
| | Nutrition/Hydration: | | |
| | Notes: | | |

| Date: | | Plan: | | |
|---|---|---|---|---|
| **WORKOUT DESCRIPTION** | Run: | Cross-Train: | | Strength: |
| | Time of Day: | Weather: | | Cycle Day: |
| | Nutrition/Hydration: | | | |
| | Notes: | | | |

| Date: | | Plan: | | |
|---|---|---|---|---|
| **WORKOUT DESCRIPTION** | Run: | Cross-Train: | | Strength: |
| | Time of Day: | Weather: | | Cycle Day: |
| | Nutrition/Hydration: | | | |
| | Notes: | | | |

| Date: | | Plan: | | |
|---|---|---|---|---|
| **WORKOUT DESCRIPTION** | Run: | Cross-Train: | | Strength: |
| | Time of Day: | Weather: | | Cycle Day: |
| | Nutrition/Hydration: | | | |
| | Notes: | | | |

| Date: | | Plan: | | |
|---|---|---|---|---|
| **WORKOUT DESCRIPTION** | Run: | Cross-Train: | | Strength: |
| | Time of Day: | Weather: | | Cycle Day: |
| | Nutrition/Hydration: | | | |
| | Notes: | | | Weekly Mileage: |

# Week #:  Trust your training!  Dates:

**How I'm Feeling:**

**Weekly Goals:**

| Date: | Plan: | |
|---|---|---|
| **WORKOUT DESCRIPTION** Run: | Cross-Train: | Strength: |
| Time of Day: | Weather: | Cycle Day: |
| Nutrition/Hydration: | | |
| Notes: | | |

| Date: | Plan: | |
|---|---|---|
| **WORKOUT DESCRIPTION** Run: | Cross-Train: | Strength: |
| Time of Day: | Weather: | Cycle Day: |
| Nutrition/Hydration: | | |
| Notes: | | |

| Date: | Plan: | |
|---|---|---|
| **WORKOUT DESCRIPTION** Run: | Cross-Train: | Strength: |
| Time of Day: | Weather: | Cycle Day: |
| Nutrition/Hydration: | | |
| Notes: | | |

| WORKOUT DESCRIPTION | Date: | | Plan: | | |
|---|---|---|---|---|---|
| | Run: | | Cross-Train: | | Strength: |
| | Time of Day: | | Weather: | | Cycle Day: |
| | Nutrition/Hydration: | | | | |
| | Notes: | | | | |

| WORKOUT DESCRIPTION | Date: | | Plan: | | |
|---|---|---|---|---|---|
| | Run: | | Cross-Train: | | Strength: |
| | Time of Day: | | Weather: | | Cycle Day: |
| | Nutrition/Hydration: | | | | |
| | Notes: | | | | |

| WORKOUT DESCRIPTION | Date: | | Plan: | | |
|---|---|---|---|---|---|
| | Run: | | Cross-Train: | | Strength: |
| | Time of Day: | | Weather: | | Cycle Day: |
| | Nutrition/Hydration: | | | | |
| | Notes: | | | | |

| WORKOUT DESCRIPTION | Date: | | Plan: | | |
|---|---|---|---|---|---|
| | Run: | | Cross-Train: | | Strength: |
| | Time of Day: | | Weather: | | Cycle Day: |
| | Nutrition/Hydration: | | | | |
| | Notes: | | | | Weekly Mileage: |

# Hydration & Nutrition Plan

On-Course Hydration & Location(s):_____

_____

On-Course Nutrition & Location(s):_____

_____

## DAYS BEFORE

Eat:_____

_____

Drink:_____

_____

## DAY/NIGHT BEFORE

Eat:_____

_____

Drink:_____

_____

## BEFORE RACE

Eat:_____

_____

_____

Drink:_____

_____

_____

## DURING RACE

Eat:_____

_____

_____

Drink:_____

_____

_____

## AFTER RACE

Eat:_____

Drink:_____

# Outfit/Costume Plan

Race Day Outfit Idea:_____

_____

_____

_____

(Sketch)

Items Needed & Plan:_____

_____

_____

_____

_____

_____

_____

_____

_____

Running Shoes/Socks/Hat/Other:_____

_____

_____

_____

_____

_____

# Travel Plan

Destination:_____

_____

_____

Travel Dates:_____

_____

_____

Names of Travelers:_____

_____

_____

_____

Transportation Plan & Information:_____

_____

_____

_____

_____

_____

_____

_____

_____

_____

_____

_____

Lodging Plan & Information:_____

_____

_____

_____

_____

_____

_____

_____

Dining Plan & Information:_____

_____
_____
_____
_____
_____
_____
_____

Daily Plan:_____

_____
_____
_____
_____
_____
_____
_____
_____
_____
_____
_____
_____
_____
_____
_____
_____
_____

Other:_____

_____
_____
_____
_____
_____
_____

# Packing List

- ☐ This Running Journal
- ☐ Expo Pass/Information
- ☐ Race Waiver/Confirmation/Bib #
- ☐ Flight & Hotel Information
- ☐ Money/Credit Card/Wallet/ID
- ☐ Cell Phone
- ☐ Emergency Contact Information
- ☐ Electronics Charger & Cords
- ☐ Sports Watch
- ☐ Glasses/Contacts/Sunglasses
- ☐ Medications/Vitamins
- ☐ Hand Sanitizer
- ☐ Hand Wipes
- ☐ Headphones
- ☐ Tissues
- ☐ Mints/Gum
- ☐ Snacks
- ☐ Water Bottle/Drink Mix
- ☐ Backpack
- ☐ Comfortable Shoes
- ☐ Jacket/Sweatshirt
- ☐ Shorts/Pants
- ☐ Shirts/Tanks/Sweaters
- ☐ Socks
- ☐ Undergarments
- ☐ Pajamas
- ☐ Swimsuit & Cover-Up
- ☐ Cold Weather Gear
- ☐ Rain Gear
- ☐ Toothbrush & Toothpaste
- ☐ Shampoo/Conditioner/Hair Care

- ☐ Razor
- ☐ Deodorant
- ☐ Lotion
- ☐ Makeup
- ☐ Nail File & Clippers
- ☐ Other Toiletries
- ☐ Race Day Breakfast
- ☐ Race Outfit
- ☐ Race Shoes
- ☐ Underwear/Sports Bra/Socks
- ☐ Running Sunglasses
- ☐ Hat/Visor/Head Band
- ☐ Extra Sports Socks
- ☐ Fitness Belt/Hydration Vest
- ☐ Sports Bottle(s)
- ☐ Race Fuel
- ☐ Race Hydration
- ☐ Throwaway Pre-Race Clothes
- ☐ Extra Race Outfit
- ☐ Gear Check Bag
- ☐ Anti-Chafe Balm
- ☐ Sunscreen
- ☐ Lip Balm
- ☐ Hair Bands
- ☐ Post-Race Clothes
- ☐ Post-Race Recovery Nutrition
- ☐ Compression Socks/Tights
- ☐ Foam Roller
- ☐ Muscle Cream
- ☐ Pain Medication
- ☐ Bandages

- ☐ _____
- ☐ _____
- ☐ _____
- ☐ _____
- ☐ _____
- ☐ _____
- ☐ _____
- ☐ _____
- ☐ _____
- ☐ _____
- ☐ _____
- ☐ _____
- ☐ _____
- ☐ _____
- ☐ _____
- ☐ _____
- ☐ _____
- ☐ _____
- ☐ _____
- ☐ _____
- ☐ _____
- ☐ _____
- ☐ _____
- ☐ _____
- ☐ _____
- ☐ _____
- ☐ _____
- ☐ _____
- ☐ _____
- ☐ _____
- ☐ _____

# To Do List

- [ ] Register for race(s)
- [ ] Add proof of time to registration
- [ ] Research and reserve flights/transportation
- [ ] Research and reserve lodging
- [ ] Create or download a training plan
- [ ] Download or print registration confirmation, race waiver, and expo pass
- [ ] _____
- [ ] _____
- [ ] _____
- [ ] _____
- [ ] _____
- [ ] _____
- [ ] _____
- [ ] _____
- [ ] _____
- [ ] _____
- [ ] _____
- [ ] _____
- [ ] _____
- [ ] _____
- [ ] _____
- [ ] _____
- [ ] _____
- [ ] _____
- [ ] _____
- [ ] _____
- [ ] _____
- [ ] _____

# Expense Tracker

| Date | Description | Cost | Method |
|------|-------------|------|--------|
|  |  |  |  |
|  |  |  |  |
|  |  |  |  |
|  |  |  |  |
|  |  |  |  |
|  |  |  |  |
|  |  |  |  |
|  |  |  |  |
|  |  |  |  |
|  |  |  |  |
|  |  |  |  |
|  |  |  |  |
|  |  |  |  |
|  |  |  |  |
|  |  |  |  |
|  |  |  |  |
|  |  |  |  |
|  |  |  |  |
|  |  |  |  |
|  |  |  |  |
|  |  |  |  |
|  |  |  |  |
|  |  |  |  |
|  |  |  |  |
|  |  |  |  |
|  |  |  |  |
|  |  |  |  |
|  | Total |  |  |

# Race Day Preparation

Week Before: _____

_____

_____

_____

_____

_____

_____

_____

Day Before: _____

_____

_____

_____

_____

_____

_____

Night Before: _____

_____

_____

_____

_____

_____

Race Morning: _____

_____

_____

_____

_____

_____

_____

_____

# Race Recap

How I Felt Before the Race: _____

_____

_____

_____

_____

_____

_____

_____

How I Felt During the Race: _____

_____

_____

_____

_____

_____

_____

_____

Things That Went Well: _____

_____

_____

_____

_____

_____

_____

_____

Things That Didn't Go Well: _____

_____

_____

_____

_____

How I Felt at the Finish: _____

_____

_____

_____

_____

_____

_____

_____

My Favorite Memories: _____

_____

_____

_____

_____

_____

_____

_____

Other Thoughts: _____

_____

_____

_____

_____

_____

My Stats: _____

_____

_____

_____

_____

# Notes:

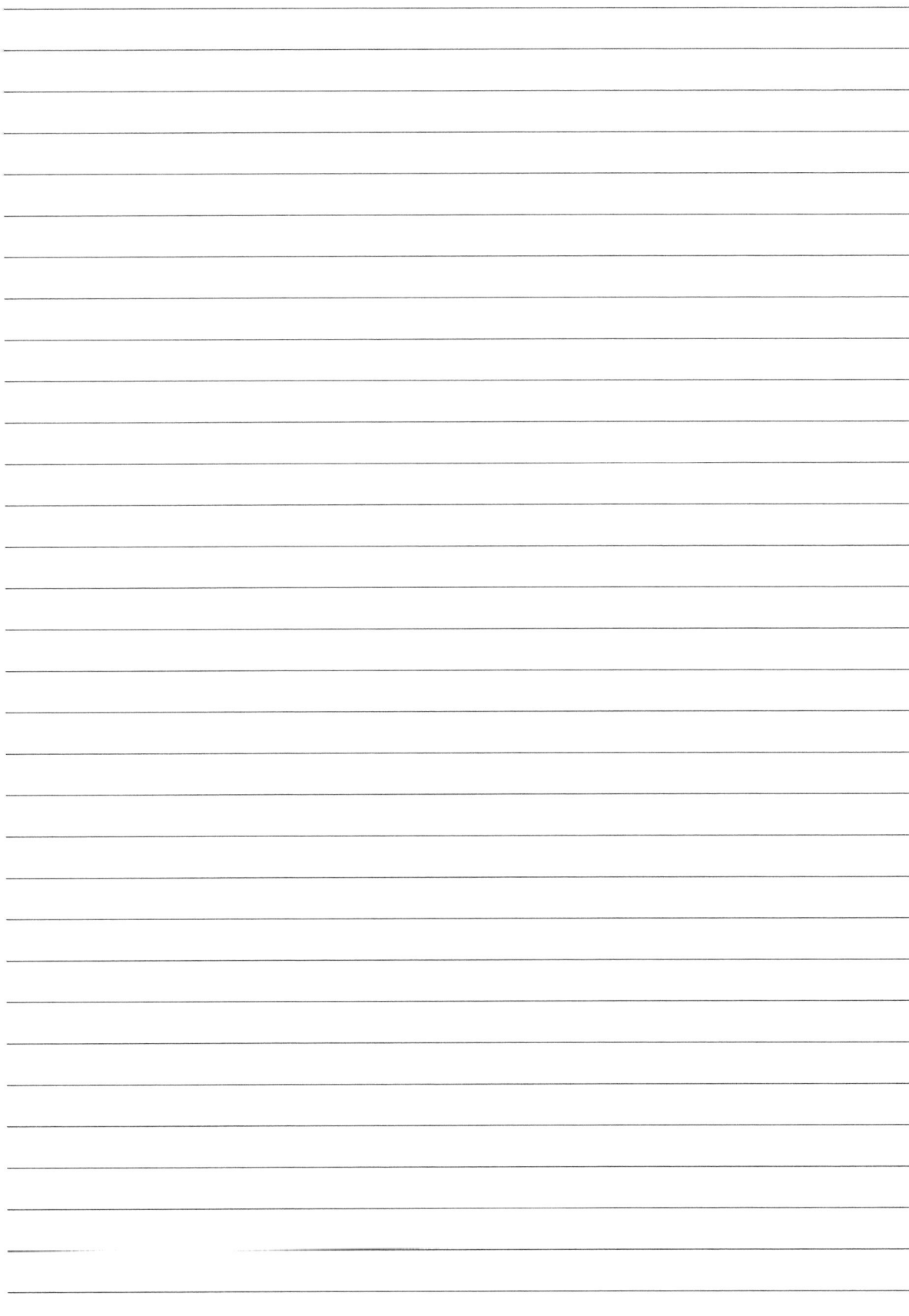

# Publisher's Note

Thank you for choosing this book!

If you like this journal, please help others find it by leaving a review online where you purchased it. If you have ideas that you would like to see included in future editions of this book, or you want to learn more about the author, visit whysheruns.com.

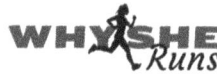

**WHY SHE** *Runs*

Enjoy your magical race!

Additional titles from this publisher:

*Word Search Puzzles for Runners: A Fun and Challenging Themed Word Search Puzzle Book for Adults, Seniors, and Teens* by Why She Runs ISBN 9798985781625

*How to Plan a Free Theme Park Vacation: Budget and Pay for Travel Using Points, Miles, and Other Rewards* by H. Kinney ISBN 9798985781618

*Theme Park Vacation Planner, Weekend Edition: A Helpful Travel Organizer to Plan and Track a Magical Trip* by H. Kinney ISBN 9798402935679

*Theme Park Vacation Planner, One-Week Edition: A Helpful Travel Organizer to Plan and Track a Magical Trip* by H. Kinney  ISBN 9798403943093

*Theme Park Vacation Planner, Two-Week Edition: A Helpful Travel Organizer to Plan and Track a Magical Trip* by H. Kinney  ISBN 9781737255772

*Looking Back and Running Forward: Discovering what it means to be broken* by Heidi Kinney ISBN 9781737255703

www.ingramcontent.com/pod-product-compliance
Lightning Source LLC
Chambersburg PA
CBHW080425030426
42335CB00020B/2592